THE NO-
PRESCRIPTION TO
REVERSING
HYPERTENSION

Copyright
@2020

Table of Contents

UNDERSTANDING HIGH BLOOD PRESSURE AND PREHYPERTENSION?

Blood pressure is the force of blood pushing against the walls of the arteries and other blood vessels. Blood pressure rises and falls throughout the day. High blood pressure is when the pressure of the blood circulating in your body stays elevated overtime and puts an excessive amount of pressure on the walls of your arteries.

This causes damage to those arteries and over time increases your risk of heart conditions and stroke. The medical term for high blood pressure is hypertension.

High blood pressure can be dangerous because it causes the heart work too hard and contributes to atherosclerosis (hardening of the arteries). It increases the risk of heart conditions and stroke, which according to statistics are the first and third leading causes of mortality among people.

High blood pressure also can result in other health conditions, like congestive heart failure, kidney disease, and blindness.

A blood pressure level of 140/90 mmHg and higher is considered high. About two-thirds of people over age 65 have hypertension. If your blood pressure is within the range of 120/80 mmHg and 139/89 mmHg, then you have prehypertension. This means that you haven't developed high blood pressure, but are quite likely to develop it in the future if you don't adopt the healthy lifestyle changes contained in this book.

Those who don't have high blood pressure at age 55 have a 90 percent chance of developing it during their lifetimes. So hypertension is a condition that most people will develop at some point in their lives.

Both numbers obtained in a blood pressure test are important, but for people above age 50, systolic pressure gives the more accurate diagnosis of high blood pressure. Systolic pressure is the number at the top in a blood pressure reading. It is considered high, when it is 140 mmHg or higher.

Category	systolic (mmHg)		diastolic (mmHg)	Remark
Normal	< 120	and	< 80	Nothing to worry about.
Elevated	120 –129	and	< 80	Your leaving the safe zone.
Prehypertension	130–139	or	80–89	You have "Stage 1" high blood pressure.
Hypertension	> 140	or	> 90	You have "Stage 2" high blood pressure.
Hypertensive Crisis	> 180	or	> 120	Critical level. See your doctor.

Recording your blood pressure makes it easier to track and control, it also provides more information for your doctor.

Search ASIN: **B0863R6BYS** on Amazon.com, and get this well-designed blood pressure logbook.

A FEW FACTS ON HIGH BLOOD PRESSURE

Hypertension is a serious health condition because it can lead to other major health problems. Make a point of learning what healthy blood pressure should be. And, remember:

- ✓ High blood pressure may not show any symptom or make you feel sick, but it is serious.
- ✓ You can lower your blood pressure by adopting a healthy day-to-day habit and by taking medicine, if needed.
- ✓ If you are taking high blood pressure medicine, making some lifestyle changes may help reduce the dose you need.
- ✓ If you take blood pressure control drugs and your blood pressure goes down, it means medicine and lifestyle changes are working for you. If another doctor asks if you have hypertension; the answer is, "Yes, but it's being treated."

✓ Tell your doctor about all the drugs you are taking. Do not forget to mention any over-the-counter drugs, vitamins, and dietary supplements. They too can affect your blood pressure, and can change the effectiveness of your blood pressure medicine.

✓ Blood pressure control pills should be taken at the same interval each day. E.g. Take your drug in the morning with breakfast or late in the evening after brushing your teeth. If you miss a dose, don't double the dose the following day.

✓ Don't take doses higher than your doctor prescribed. Do not stop taking your medicine even after you achieve a lowered blood pressure, unless your doctor directs you to stop. Don't skip doses or take half a pill. Always remember to refill your pills before the last one. If you cannot afford your medicines, discuss it with your doctor or pharmacist.

✓ Before having surgery, ask your doctor if it is safe to take your blood pressure control pill on that day.

✓ Rise slowly from a seated or lying position and stand for some seconds before walking. This allows your blood pressure adjust, to prevent fainting, dizziness, or a fall.

✓ As you get older, high blood pressure, especially isolated systolic hypertension, is more common and may increase your risk of other serious health problems. Treatment, especially if you are suffering from other medical conditions, often requires continuous evaluation and discussions with your doctor to strike the best balance of maintaining a good quality of life and reducing risks.

If your doctor directs you to take your blood pressure readings at home, keep in mind:

- ✓ There are several brands of home blood pressure monitors on sale. Confirm from your doctor, nurse, or pharmacist on which monitor you need and how to use it. Check your monitor at the doctor's office to be sure it works correctly.
- ✓ Avoid smoking, exercise, and caffeine 30 minutes before checking your blood pressure.
- ✓ Make sure you're sitting with feet uncrossed, feet on the floor, and with your back is resting against something.
- ✓ Relax perfectly for 5 minutes before checking your blood pressure.
- ✓ Keep a record of your blood pressure readings, what time you measured it, and when you took your pressure pill (if you take it). Share the recorded information with your doctor, or nurse.

HOW YOU CAN PREVENT OR CONTROL HIGH BLOOD PRESSURE?

If you have hypertension, you and your health care provider must work together as a team to lower it. The two of you need to agree on a blood pressure goal. Together, you should devise a strategy and timetable for achieving your goal.

Blood pressure is mostly measured in millimeters of mercury (mmHg) and recorded as two numbers; systolic pressure (as the heart beats) "over" diastolic pressure (as the heart relaxes between beats). For example, 130/80 mmHg.

It is always helpful to monitor your blood pressure at home between visits to your doctor. You also may want to bring a relative with you when you visit your doctor. Having a family member who is aware that you have hypertension and who understands what you need to do to get it lowered, often makes it easier to implement the changes that will help you reach your goal.

The steps listed in this book will help lower your blood pressure. If you have prehypertension, following these steps will help prevent you from developing high blood pressure.

This guide is meant to assist you adopt a healthier lifestyle and control your blood pressure naturally, without needing any drug. And to help remember to take prescribed pills, should you resort to that.

Following the steps described will facilitate your prevention and control of high blood pressure. While you read them, think on how each point applies to you, and how to put it in practice.

- Keep a healthy weight.
- Exercise every day.
- Follow a healthy eating plan.
- Cut down on sodium (salt and other sodium compound).
- Drink alcohol only moderately and don't smoke.
- Take prescribed drugs as directed.

MAINTAIN HEALTHY WEIGHT

Being overweight or obese increases the risk of developing high blood pressure. In fact, your blood pressure rises as you gain body weight. Losing even 10 pounds can significantly lower your blood pressure; and losing weight has the highest effectiveness on those who are overweight and have already developed hypertension.

Overweight and obesity also are risk factors for heart disease. Being overweight or obese raises your chances of developing diabetes and high blood cholesterol; two more risk factors for heart disease.

Two key measures can be used to determine if someone is overweight or obese. These are body mass index (BMI), and waist circumference.

BMI is a measure of the body weight relative to height. It gives an approximation of total body fat, and that is what multiplies the risk of diseases that are related to being overweight.

Relying on BMI alone doesn't determine risk. For example, in someone who is very muscular or who has swelling from fluid retention (edema), BMI may overestimate body fat. BMI may underestimate body fat in older persons or those losing muscle.

That's why waist measurement is usually checked as well. Another reason is that excessive fat in the stomach area also increases disease risk. A waist measurement higher than 35 inches in women and 40 inches in men is considered high.

Height	Body Weight (lb)										
4'10"	100	105	110	115	119	124	129	134	138	143	148
5'0"	107	112	118	123	128	133	138	143	148	153	158
5'2"	115	120	126	131	136	142	147	153	158	164	169
5'4"	122	128	134	140	145	151	157	163	169	174	180
5'6"	130	136	142	148	155	161	167	173	179	186	192
5'8"	138	144	151	158	164	171	177	184	190	197	203
5'10"	146	153	160	167	174	181	188	195	202	209	216
6'0"	154	162	169	177	184	191	199	206	213	221	228
6'2"	163	171	179	186	194	202	210	218	225	233	241
6'4"	172	180	189	197	205	213	221	320	238	246	254
BMI	21	22	23	24	25	26	27	28	29	30	31

Check the chart above to find your corresponding approximate healthy BMI value. And also, the chat bellow to determine if you are at a normal weight, overweight, or obese. Overweight is defined as a BMI of 25 to 29.9; obesity is defined as a BMI equal to or higher than 30.

If you fall within the obese range according to the guidelines in the chat, you're at increased risk for heart disease and you are advised to lose weight. You also should consider losing weight if you have two or more heart disease risk factors.

If you fall within the normal weight range or are overweight but don't need to lose weight, but still take measures not to gain more weight.

Here is a chart that groups BMI for various heights and weights

CATEGORY	BMI	REMARK
Normal Weight	18.5 – 24.9	Your form is good. Try not to gain weight.
Overweight	25 – 29.9	Do not gain any weight, especially if your waist measurement is high. You need to lose weight if you have two or more risk factors for heart disease.
Obese	30 or >30	You need to lose weight. Lose weight slowly; about 1/2 pound to 2 pounds a week.

If you need to lose weight, it's important to take it slowly. Do not lose more than 1/2 pound to 2 pounds in a week. You may start with a goal of losing 10 percent of your current weight. This is often the healthiest way to drop some weight and offers the best chance of long-term success.

There's no magic formula for weight loss. You have to eat significantly less calories than you use up in daily activities. The amount of calories you burn daily depends on body size and level of physically activities.

One pound equals 3,500 calories. So, to lose 1 pound in a week, you need to eat 500 calories a day less or burn 500 calories a day more than you usually do. It's best to devise some combination of both eating less and being more physically active. Remember to mind the serving sizes. It's not only what you eat, but also how much.

EXERCISE EVERY DAY

Being physically active is among the most important things you can do to control or prevent high blood pressure. It also helps to reduce your risk of heart disease.

It doesn't require plenty of effort to become physically active. All it takes is 30 minutes of moderate-level physical activity on every or most days of the week. Examples of such activities are bicycling, raking leaves, road walks and gardening.

You can even divide the half-hour into shorter periods of at least 10 minutes each. E.g. Get off a bus one or two stops early, use stairs instead of an elevator, or park your car at the far end of the lot at work. If you already engage in 30 minutes of moderate-level physical activity a day, you can get added benefits by doing more. Engage in a moderate-level activity for a longer period each day or more vigorous activity for a shorter time.

Most people don't need to see a doctor before they start to engage in daily moderate-level physical activity. You should discuss first with your doctor if you have heart condition or have had a heart attack, if you're over 50years and are not used to moderate-level physical activity, if you have a family history of heart disease at young age, or if you have other serious health condition.

Common Chores	Sporting Activities
Gardening for 45 minutes	Bicycling 5 miles in 30minutes
Shoveling snow for 15 minutes	Swimming for 20 minutes
Stair walking for 15 minutes	Skip rope for 15 minutes
Carry a 25Kg log for half a mile under 20 minutes	Playing volleyball for an hour
	Playing basketball for 20 minutes

FOLLOW A HEALTHY DIET PLAN

Your choice of food affects your chances of developing high blood pressure. A healthy diet plan can both reduce the risk of having high blood pressure and lower a blood pressure that is already too high.

For an overall eating plan, consider DASH, which stands for "Dietary Approaches to Stop Hypertension." You can lower your blood pressure by eating foods that have low saturated fat, total fat, and cholesterol, and rich in fruits, vegetables, and low-fat dairy foods. The DASH diet plan includes whole grains, nuts, fish, and poultry, and has low amounts of fats, sweets, red meats, sodium compounds, and sugared beverages. It is also high in potassium, magnesium, and calcium, as well as protein and fiber. Eating foods lower in salt and sodium is known to reduce blood pressure.

The table below gives the servings and food groups for the DASH eating plan. The amount of servings that is right for you may vary, depending on individual caloric need.

The DASH eating plan has more daily servings of fruits, vegetables, and grains than you may be used to eating. Those foods are high in fiber, and consuming more of them may temporarily cause bloating and diarrhea. To get used to the DASH eating plan, gradually increase your servings of grains, fruits, and vegetables.

A more convenient way to switch to the DASH eating plan is to keep a record of your current eating habits. Write down what you eat, when, how much, and why. Note whether you snack on high-fat foods while watching television or if you skip breakfast and eat a big lunch. Do this for several days and you will be able to figure where you can start making changes.

If you're trying to slim down, you should choose a diet plan that is lower in calories. You can still use the DASH diet plan, but follow it at a lower calorie level. Again, a food diary may be helpful. It can tell you if there are certain times that you eat without feeling really hungry or when you can substitute low-calorie foods for high-calorie foods.

The DASH eating plan shown below is based on 2,000 calories a day. The number of daily servings in a food group may vary from those listed, depending upon your caloric needs.

Food Group	Daily Servings	Serving Sizes
Grains and grain products	7-8	1 slice bread 1 cup ready-to-eat cereal $^1/_2$ cup cooked rice, pasta, or cereal
Vegetables	4-5	1 cup raw leafy vegetable $^1/_2$ cup cooked vegetable 6 ounces vegetable juice
Fruits	4-5	1 medium fruit (E.g. mango, orange or apple) $^1/_4$ cup dried fruit $^1/_2$ cup fresh, frozen, or canned fruit 6 ounces fruit juice
Low-fat or fat free dairy foods	2-3	8 ounces milk 1 cup yogurt 1 $^1/_2$ ounces cheese
Lean meats, poultry, and fish	2 or fewer	3 ounces cooked lean meat, skinless poultry, or fish
Nuts, seeds, and dry beans	4-5 per week	$^1/_3$ cup or 1 $^1/_2$ ounces nuts 1 tablespoon or $^1/_2$ ounce seeds $^1/_2$ cup cooked dry beans
Fats and oils	2-3	1 teaspoon soft margarine 1 tablespoon low-fat mayonnaise 2 tablespoons light salad dressing 1 teaspoon vegetable oil
Sweets	5 per week	1 tablespoon sugar 1 tablespoon jelly or jam $^1/_2$ ounce jelly beans 8 ounces lemonade

The DASH eating plan was not original designed to promote weight loss. But it is rich in low-calorie foods such as fruits and vegetables. You can further lower the calorie content by replacing high-calorie foods with more fruits and vegetables; and that also will hasten your journey to reach your DASH eating plan goals. Here are some examples.

To increase fruits:

- Eat a medium apple instead of four shortbread cookies. You'll save 80 calories.
- Eat $\frac{1}{4}$ cup of dried apricots instead of a 2-ounce bag of pork rinds. You'll save 230 calories.

To increase vegetables:

- Have a hamburger that's 3 ounces instead of 6 ounces. Add a $\frac{1}{2}$ cup serving of spinach and a $\frac{1}{2}$ cup serving of carrots. You'll save more than 200 calories.
- Instead of 5 ounces of chicken, have a stir fry with 2 ounces of chicken and $1\frac{1}{2}$ cups of raw vegetables. Use a small amount of vegetable oil. You'll save 50 calories.

To increase low-fat or fat free dairy products:

- Have a $^1/_2$ cup serving of low-fat frozen yogurt instead of a $1^1/_2$ ounce milk chocolate bar. You'll save about 110 calories.

And don't forget these calorie-saving tips:

- Use low-fat or fat free condiments, such as fat free salad dressings.
- Eat smaller portions—cut back gradually.
- Choose low-fat or fat free dairy products to reduce total fat intake.
- Use food labels to compare fat content in packaged foods. Items labelled low-fat or fat free are not always lower in calories than their regular versions. I've added a guide on how to read and compare food labels. You'll find it as you read.
- Limit foods with lots of added sugar, such as pies, flavored yogurts, candy bars, ice cream, sherbet, regular soft drinks, and fruit drinks.
- Eat fruits canned in their own juice.

- Snack on fruit, vegetable sticks, unbuttered and unsalted popcorn, or bread sticks.
- Drink water or club soda.

MORE SPICE AND LESS SALT

An important part of healthy eating is choosing foods that are low in salt (sodium chloride) and other forms of sodium compound. Consuming less sodium is key to maintaining blood pressure at a healthy level.

Most people use more salt and sodium than they need. Some people, such as African-American and the elderly, are especially sensitive to salt and sodium and should be particularly careful about how much they consume.

Most people should consume no more than 2.4 grams (2,400 milligrams) of sodium a day. That equals 6 grams (about 1 teaspoon) of table salt a day. For someone with hypertension, the doctor may advise less. The 6 grams includes all salt and sodium consumed in other forms, including that used in cooking and at the table.

Before trying salt substitutes, you should inquire from your doctor, especially if you have high blood pressure. These contain potassium chloride and may be unsafe for those with certain medical conditions.

Tips to reduce sodium

- ✓ Use herbs, spices, and salt-free seasoning blends in cooking and at the table.
- ✓ Buy fresh, plain frozen, or canned "with no salt added" vegetables.
- ✓ Use fresh fish, poultry, and lean meat, rather than canned or processed types.
- ✓ Choose ready-to-eat breakfast cereals that are low in sodium. If you can avoid read-to-eat foods
- ✓ Choose "convenience" foods that contain low sodium. Cut back on frozen dinners, pizza, salad dressings, packaged mixes, and canned soups or broths—these often contain a lot of sodium.
- ✓ Cook rice, pasta, and hot cereal without salt. Cut back on instant or flavored rice, pasta, and cereal mixes, which usually have added salt.
- ✓ Always rinse canned foods, such as tuna, to remove some sodium.
- ✓ Buy low or reduced-sodium or no-salt-added versions of foods, when available.

With herbs, spices, onion, and garlic, you can make your food spicy without adding salt and sodium. There's no reason why eating less sodium should make your food any less delicious! Check the following chat for some awesome ideas on using herbs and spices.

Herbs and Spices	Usage
Ginger	Soups, salads, vegetables, and meats
Dill (Weed and Seed)	Fish, soups, salads, and vegetables
Cloves	Soups, salads, and vegetables
Chili Powder	Soups, salads, vegetables, and fish
Cinnamon	Salads, vegetables, breads, and snacks
Basil	Soups and salads, vegetables, fish, and meats
Thyme	Salads, vegetables, fish, and chicken
Sage	Soups, salads, vegetables, meats, and chicken
Rosemary	Salads, vegetables, fish, and meats
Parsley	Salads, vegetables, fish, and meats
Oregano	Soups, salads, vegetables, meats, and snacks
Nutmeg	Vegetables, meats, and snacks
Marjoram	Soups, salads, vegetables, beef, fish, and chicken

Experiment with these and other herbs and spices. To start, use small amounts to know if you like them.

Pay Attention to Food Label

By paying close attention to labels when you shop for food, you can consume less sodium. Sodium is found naturally in many foods. But processed foods account for most of the salt and sodium that is consumed. Processed foods that contain high amount of salt include regular canned vegetables and soups, lunchmeats, frozen dinners, instant and ready-to-eat cereals, and salty chips and other snacks.

Use food labels to help you choose products that are low in sodium. The illustration bellow shows you how to read and compare food labels.

As you read food labels, you may be surprised to discover that many foods contain sodium, including baking soda, monosodium glutamate (MSG), soy sauce, seasoned salts, and some antacids.

The bellow label comparison shows that canned peas have three times more sodium than the frozen peas. That makes the frozen peas a better option.

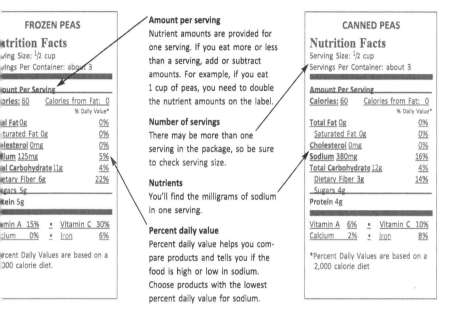

FROZEN PEAS

itrition Facts
ing Size: 1/2 cup
ings Per Container: about 3

ount Per Serving		
ries: 60	Calories from Fat: 0	
		% Daily Value*
al Fat 0g		0%
turated Fat 0g		0%
lesterol 0mg		0%
ium 125mg		5%
al Carbohydrate 11g		4%
etary Fiber 6g		22%
gars 5g		
tein 5g		

| min A 15% | • | Vitamin C 30% |
| cium 0% | • | Iron 6% |

rcent Daily Values are based on a
000 calorie diet.

Amount per serving
Nutrient amounts are provided for one serving. If you eat more or less than a serving, add or subtract amounts. For example, if you eat 1 cup of peas, you need to double the nutrient amounts on the label.

Number of servings
There may be more than one serving in the package, so be sure to check serving size.

Nutrients
You'll find the milligrams of sodium in one serving.

Percent daily value
Percent daily value helps you compare products and tells you if the food is high or low in sodium. Choose products with the lowest percent daily value for sodium.

CANNED PEAS

Nutrition Facts
Serving Size: 1/2 cup
Servings Per Container: about 3

Amount Per Serving		
Calories: 60	Calories from Fat: 0	
		% Daily Value*
Total Fat 0g		0%
Saturated Fat 0g		0%
Cholesterol 0mg		0%
Sodium 380mg		16%
Total Carbohydrate 12g		4%
Dietary Fiber 3g		14%
Sugars 4g		
Protein 4g		

| Vitamin A 6% | • | Vitamin C 10% |
| Calcium 2% | • | Iron 8% |

*Percent Daily Values are based on a 2,000 calorie diet

More tips to keep in mind

✓ Vegetables and fruit are naturally low in sodium

✓ Eat fewer packaged, ready-to-eat and take-out foods

✓ At home, prepare your own meals often, or have them prepered by someone who understands your health condition and your goal.

27

- ✓ Flavour your foods with herbs and salt-free spices, garlic, vinegar, lemon, lime, ginger and onion
- ✓ Rinse and drain canned vegetables and canned beans, peas and lentils under cold, running water
- ✓ Taste your food before adding any salt, you may discover you don't need to
- ✓ Use the % Daily Value (%DV) on the food label to check if a food contains little or a lot of sodium. Choose products with a sodium content of less than 15% DV
- ✓ When eating out, pay attention to the nutritional information of menu items and choose foods with less sodium. You can also request for your food to be made without salt or monosodium glutamate (MSG) and to have salty sauces, dressings, and condiments served on the side or separately.

Garlic, thyme, and Aloe Vera are particularly effective in lowering blood pressure.

REDUCE OR AVOID ALCHOHOL AND DON'T SMOKE

Drinking too much alcohol can raise blood pressure. It also can harm the heart, liver, and brain. Alcoholic drinks also contain calories, which defeats your efforts if you are trying to lose weight. Smoking increases the risk of developing high blood pressure, and other serious health problems. If you smoke, quit.

If you drink alcoholic beverages, drink only a moderate amount:

- o **For men:** fewer than 15 drinks per week, with no more than 2 drinks a day on most days
- o **For women:** fewer than 10 drinks per week, with no more than 2 drinks a day on most days

What counts as a drink?	
Alcohol Type	Amount
Liquor – 40% alcohol content (e.g. rum, rye, vodka, gin)	43 mL (1.5 oz), 100 calories
Wine – 12% alcohol content	148 mL (5 oz), 100 calories
Beer, cider, or cooler – 5% alcohol content	355 mL (12 oz), 150 calories

HERBS THAT WORK

- **Cinnamon:** is another tasty seasoning that requires little effort to include in your daily diet. One study done in rodents suggested that cinnamon extract lowered both sudden and prolonged high blood pressure. However, the extract was administered intravenously. It's unclear if cinnamon consumed orally is also effective.

  You would have to consume cinnamon in very high doses to experience any worrisome side effect.

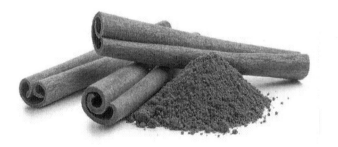

Cinnamon and diabetes:

Some smaller studies prove that cinnamon does have an effect on blood glucose levels in those with Type-

2 Diabetes. Interestingly, there seems to be a different effect based on the type of cinnamon used. The Cassia cinnamon has shown the most promise in the control of blood glucose, while the Ceylon species of cinnamon is just beginning to be studied. This may be partially because Ceylon is harder to come by than Cassia.

Another smaller Chinese study published in the journal Nutrition Research found evidence of cinnamon lowering blood glucose levels in patients that took cinnamon supplements, in contrast to those who were given a placebo.

Cinnamon has also been shown to lower the cholesterol levels of patients with diabetes.

Cinnamon and weight loss:

Cinnamon has been shown to reduce some of the bad effects of eating high-fat foods. This can help in an overall weight loss plan. Its effect on blood glucose levels can also help your body ultimately lose weight.

The anti-inflammatory and antibacterial properties of cinnamon can provide additional help to those trying to lose weight by promoting an overall healthy body that'll process food better.

It is important to note that cinnamon alone will not lead to long-term weight loss. But it would be beneficial to add cinnamon to your healthy diet and exercise plan to help you reach your weight loss goal. One teaspoon of cinnamon does contain 1.6 grams of fiber, which can help you reach your daily fiber goal and increase a feeling of fullness at meals.

Other health benefits of cinnamon:

Studies have shown that a variety of other medical conditions can be improved (or in some way positively affected) through the use of cinnamon.

Some of these include:

- o   Alzheimer's
- o   HIV

- o Multiple Sclerosis

- o Chronic Wounds

- o Digestive Problems

- o Respiratory illness

- o Gynecological Issues

- **Holy Basil** (*Ocimum tenuiflorum*): is a delicious herb that goes well in a variety of foods. This green leafy plant might help lower your blood pressure. The chemical eugenol, which is found in basil, may block certain substances that tighten blood vessels. This may lead to a drop in blood pressure. In a study, basil extract has been shown to lower blood pressure in rodents, although only briefly.

  Adding fresh basil to your diet is easy and certainly can't hurt. Keep a small pot of the herb in your kitchen garden and add the fresh leaves to pastas, soups, salads, and casseroles.

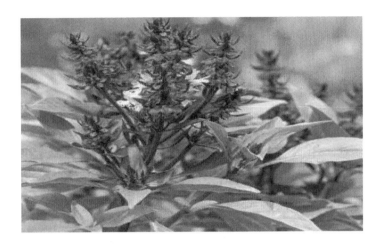

Other common uses of Holy Basil

From the leaves to the seed, holy basil is considered a tonic for the body, mind, and spirit. Different parts of the plant are effective in treating different conditions:

- o Use the ointment form for eczema.
- o Use an alcohol extract for stomach ulcers and eye diseases.
- o Use its fresh flowers for bronchitis.
- o Use the leaves and seeds, with black pepper, for malaria.

- o Use the whole plant for diarrhea, nausea, and vomiting.

- o Use an essential oil made from the leaves for insect bites.

Many studies support the use of the entire plant of holy basil for human use and its therapeutic value.

The **nutritional value** is also high, as it contains: Vitamin A and C, Calcium, Zinc, Iron, Chlorophyll.

Always talk to your doctor before taking supplements. Like many supplements, holy basil is not approved as a first-line treatment. It may also interact with medications you're already taking.

- • **Celery seed:** is an herb used to flavor soups, stews, casseroles, and other savory dishes. Celery has long been used to treat hypertension in China, and studies have shown that it may be effective. You can use the seeds, or you can juice the whole plant. The juice will add a wealth of nutrient to your body. It's refreshing, contains low calories but yet gives energy.

Celery may also be a diuretic, which may help explain its effect on blood pressure. ResearchersTrusted Source believe that a variety of substances in celery may play a role in lowering blood pressure. However, human studies have not been done.

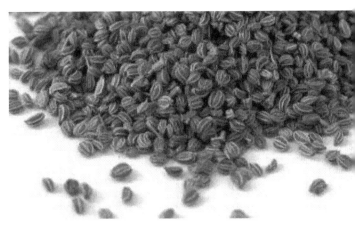

Celery juice nutrition: One glass of celery juice only contains about 40 calories, and the following important nutrients:

- ✓ Vitamins A, K, And C

- ✓ Beta Carotene

- ✓ Flavonoids

- ✓ Phytonutrients

- ✓ Calcium

- ✓ Iron

- ✓ Magnesium

- ✓ Phosphorus

- ✓ Potassium

- **French Lavender:** The beautiful color, and perfume-like scent of lavender is not the only useful aspect of the plant. Lavender extracts have been shown to lower heart rate and blood pressure in rodents. Although not many people think to use lavender as a culinary herb, you can use the flowers in baked goods. The leaves can be used in the same way you would use rosemary.

Lavender

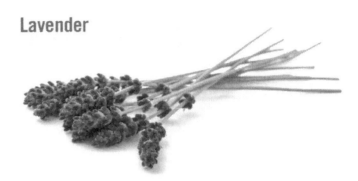

Lavender is also effective in the treatment of other health conditions. Such as: cancer, headaches, depression, anxiety, mental issues, insomnia, toothache, nausea, hair loss, acne and skin irritations.

- **Cat's Claw:** is an herbal medicine used in traditional Chinese practice to treat hypertension as well as neurological health problems.

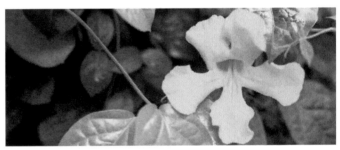

Experiments of Cat's Claw on rodents as a treatment for hypertension indicate that it may be helpful in reducing blood pressure by interfering with calcium channels in the cells. Cat's Claw is available in supplement form from many health foods stores.

- **Cardamom:** is a seasoning that comes from India and is often used in South Asian cuisine, with an intense sweet flavor, known to lower blood pressure, improve breathing and aid weight loss. A study carried on a small group of 20 adults who were diagnosed with high blood pressure to investigate the health effects of cardamom, found that participants with high blood pressure recorded significant reductions in their blood pressure readings, after taking 1.5 grams of cardamom powder twice daily for 12 weeks. Cardamom seeds or powder can be added in spice rubs, soups and stews, and even baked goods for a special flavor and a possible positive health benefit. Another good new is that cardamom is safe for most people and widely available.

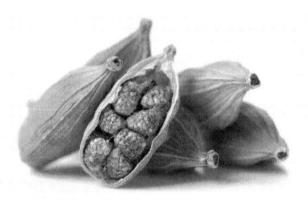

Other health benefits of cardamom:

Due to its high antioxidant and diuretic properties, cardamom may be helpful in the treatment of health conditions such as:

- o **Cancer and tumor:** Certain compounds in cardamom may fight cancer and stop the growth of tumors.
- o **Chronic diseases:** The antioxidant compound in cardamom can help protect cells from damage, stall and prevent inflammations.
- o **Antibacterial:** Extracts of cardamom proves effective against a variety of bacterial strains that cause various types of infections.

- **Flax seed:** is rich in omega-3 fatty acids, and has been shown in some studies to lower blood pressure. A recent review suggested taking 30–50 grams of whole or ground seeds daily for more than 12 weeks to get the best benefits. Flax seed may protect against atherosclerotic cardiovascular disease by reducing serum cholesterol, improving glucose tolerance, and acting as an antioxidant.

You can buy many products that contain flax seed, but a better bet is to buy whole or ground flax seed and add it to your home-cooked meals. The best part about flax seed is that it can be stirred into virtually any dish, from soups to smoothies to baked goods. Storing flax seed in your freezer may help it retain optimum potency.

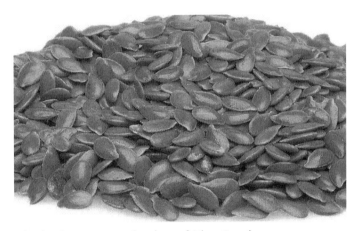

The high nutritional value of Flax Seeds:

Just one tablespoon (7 grams) which is the typical serving size; provides a good amount of protein, fiber and omega-3 fatty acids, in addition to being a rich source of some vitamins and minerals.

One tablespoon of ground flax seeds contains the following:

- ✓ Calories: 37
- ✓ Protein: 1.3 grams
- ✓ Carbs: 2 grams
- ✓ Fiber: 1.9 grams
- ✓ Total fat: 3 grams

- ✓ Saturated fat: 0.3 grams
- ✓ Monounsaturated fat: 0.5 grams
- ✓ Polyunsaturated fat: 2.0 grams
- ✓ Omega-3 fatty acids: 1,597 mg
- ✓ Vitamin B1: 8% of the RDI
- ✓ Vitamin B6: 2% of the RDI
- ✓ Folate: 2% of the RDI
- ✓ Calcium: 2% of the RDI
- ✓ Iron: 2% of the RDI
- ✓ Magnesium: 7% of the RDI
- ✓ Phosphorus: 4% of the RDI
- ✓ Potassium: 2% of the RDI

Interestingly, the health benefits of flax seeds are mainly attributed to the omega-3 fatty acids, lignans and fiber they contain.

- **Garlic:** The Cleveland Clinic puts this pungent seasoning on its list of 36 power foods, because it can do more than just flavor your food and ruin your breath. Garlic may have the ability to lower your blood pressure by helping to increase a substance in the body known as nitric oxide, which can cause your blood vessels to relax and dilate. This lets blood flow more freely and reduces blood pressure.

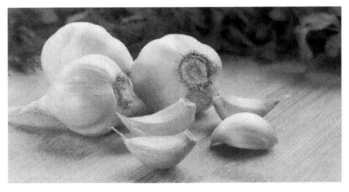

Garlic is rich in phytochemicals that are thought to ward off disease. The power in this clove is also effective in the treatment of high cholesterol, heart disease, and various types of cancer.

- **Ginger:** being among the healthiest spices on the planet; loaded with nutrients and bioactive compounds that have immense benefits for your body and brain, it can help control blood pressure also. In animal studies it has been shown to improve blood circulation and relax the muscles surrounding blood vessels, lowering blood pressure. Human studies so far have been inconclusive. Commonly used in Asian foods, ginger is a versatile ingredient that can also be added to sweets or beverages.

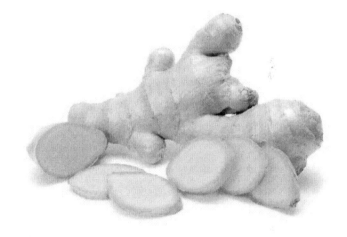

Ginger has a long history of use in the prevention and treatment of many health problems such as: inflammations, nausea, osteoarthritis, indigestion, menstrual pain, cancer, Alzheimer's disease, and high cholesterol.

- **Hawthorn:** is an herbal remedy for high blood pressure that has been used in traditional Chinese medicines for thousands of years.

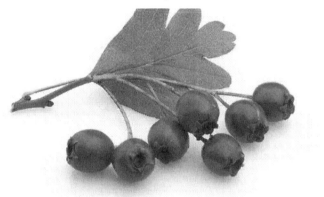

  The extracts of hawthorn seem to have a whole host of benefits on cardiovascular health, including helping reduce blood pressure, preventing hardening of the arteries, and lowering cholesterol. You can take hawthorn as a pill, liquid extract, or tea.

USING DRUGS

If you have high blood pressure, the lifestyle habits noted above may not lower your blood pressure enough. If they don't, you'll need to take drugs.

Even if you need drugs, you still must make the lifestyle changes. Doing so will help your drugs work better and may reduce how much of them you need.

There are many drugs available to lower blood pressure. They work in various ways. Most people need to take two or more drugs to bring their blood pressure down to a healthy level.

High blood pressure main types of drugs and how they work

Drug Category	How They Work
Diuretic	These are sometimes called "water pills" because they work in the kidney and flush excess water and sodium from the body through urine.
Beta-blockers	These reduce nerve impulses to the heart and blood vessels. This makes the heart beat less

	often and with less force. As a result, blood pressure drops, and the heart works less hard.
Angiotensin converting enzyme inhibitors	These inhibit the formation of a hormone called angiotensin II, which normally makes blood vessels to narrow. The blood vessels relax, and pressure goes down.
Angiotensin antagonists	These shield blood vessels from angiotensin II. As a result, the blood vessels open wider, and pressure goes down.
Calcium channel blockers	These keep calcium from entering the muscle cells of the heart and blood vessels. Blood vessels relax, and pressure goes down.
Alpha-blockers	These reduce nerve impulses to blood vessels, allowing blood to pass more easily
Alpha-beta-blockers	These work the same way as alpha-blockers but also slow the heartbeat, as beta-blockers do.
Nervous system inhibitors	These relax blood vessels by controlling nerve impulses.
Vasodilators	These directly open blood vessels by relaxing the muscle in the vessel walls.

When opting for high blood pressure control drugs, discuss with your doctor to get the particular drug and dose level that is right for you. If you begin to experience side effects, tell your doctor so the drugs can be adjusted. If you're worried about the cost of the prescribed pills, tell your doctor or pharmacist—there may be a less expensive alternative or a generic form that you can use instead.

It's important that you take your drugs as prescribed. That can prevent stroke, heart attack, and congestive heart failure, which is a critical condition in which the heart does not pump as much blood as the body requires.

Sometimes, it's easy to forget to take medicines. But just like putting your socks on in the morning and brushing your teeth, you can make your medicine become part of your daily routine. I have included some tips that will help you remember to duly take your blood pressure drugs.

Tips to help you remember to take your drugs

✓ Paste favorite picture of yourself or a loved one on the door of the refrigerator or any locker you access often, with a note next to it that says, "Remember to Take Your High Blood Pressure Drugs."

✓ Keep your high blood pressure pills on the nightstand next to your side of the bed.

✓ Keep your high blood pressure drugs with your toothbrush as a reminder. So, you take them right after you brush your teeth.

✓ Paste "sticky notes" in visible places as a reminder to take your high blood pressure drugs. You can put notes on the bathroom mirror, or on the front door.

✓ Agree with a friend who also is on daily medication to call each other every day with a reminder to "take your respective drugs."

✓ Little ones love to help the grown-ups. Ask your child or grandchild to call you every day with a quick reminder. It's also a great way to stay in touch.

✓ If you have a personal computer, program a start-up reminder to take your high blood pressure drugs, or set a daily reminder on your mobile phone to always beep at the time you are due to take your drug.

✓ Remember to refill your prescription. Each time you pick up a refill, make a reminder on your calendar to order and pick up the next refill 1 week before the medication is due to run out.

You can be taking prescribed drugs and still not have your blood pressure under control. Everyone and older people in particular, must be careful to keep his or her blood pressure below 140/90 mmHg. If your blood pressure is higher than that, discuss with your doctor about adjusting your prescription or making lifestyle changes to lower your blood pressure.

Some over-the-counter drugs, such as arthritis and pain drugs, and dietary supplements, such as ephedra, bitter orange, and ma haung, can raise your blood pressure. Be sure to inform your doctor about any nonprescription drugs that you take and ask how they may interfere with your blood pressure.

Please, give this book an honest review.

Printed in Poland
by Amazon Fulfillment
Poland Sp. z o.o., Wrocław

58954310R00035